A Collection of Reader-Submitted Medical Stories

Kerry Hamm

Copyright © 2017
All Rights Reserved.

Disclaimer:

Names, locations, and portions of the details included in this book have been altered to protect the privacy of those involved.

By now, I am sure you are all too familiar with my *Real Stories from a Small-Town ER* series, which were collections of stories told to you from my time as a registration clerk in Ohio. If you are new here, don't fret! You don't have to worry about a 'certain order' for *any* of my books, including this one!

I have since moved on from the hospital scene, but that hasn't stopped readers from submitting stories of their own experiences from the medical field. Over time, I have received hundreds of stories-some funny, some sad, some downright scary or grotesque- and have worked with my readers to bring these stories to you in a follow up to my last *Real Stories* volume.

If I've learned anything from writing my series and compiling this book, it's that none of us are alone. We're all proof that we've seen some seriously messed up things out there, right? We have seen the good. We've seen the bad. We've seen the downright vile and disgusting. And then, we've seen the humor in these situations and we've been fortunate enough to share them with one another. There is a certain peace in knowing that as no matter how crazy we feel, we have formed solidarity amongst ourselves, knowing that for every bad day you've had, others have had them too. We have worked through the challenges of getting up and facing another drug seeker, another child abuse case, another young death, and another 'how the heck did that even happen?' moment together. You guys are not alone, and this book reaffirms that.

Several of the stories have been edited to bring you clear-cut and clean versions of tales submitted by loyal readers. I have done my very best to edit out hospital and town names, and in some cases my submitters wished to withhold their initials and other details from publication or requested that I edit stories for grammar/spelling. Some stories have been edited for length. I do my very best to preserve a reader's humor and emotions, as well as capture the reader's personality when I edit these submissions.

Though some of the stories in this collection are horrifying, I am glad none of us are alone in what we've witnessed or experienced.

Suggested Serving Size

During my busy day shift at one of several emergency rooms in this city, a man ran inside, stopped in the lobby, and screamed to a room of roughly sixty people, "Someone needs to help my wife. She can't get it out!"

The man then ran back outside, where he paced the parking lot and hoped someone would follow.

I called one of our triage nurses to the front and thought she was going to smack the brain right out of my head because I couldn't tell her exactly what we were expecting. We were backed up, with six-hour waiting times, so the nurse told me to call her when the patient was inside, only if the complaint was serious.

Two armed security guards went to the parking lot to find out what we were facing.

One of the guards radioed the guard at our registration window. Through the guard's choking laughter, every last patient in our nearby Fast Track rooms, all three registration clerks, and two nurses heard, "You guys really need to see this. I've never seen anything like it before."

I was new and I was nervous. My coworkers were excited.

The security guard asked us to send a nurse and a gurney, as the female was unable to sit or walk. Two nurses who were chit-chatting in our office grumbled but complied.

I don't know why the nurses didn't use the side entrance for this patient, but I'm assuming her attitude had much to do about that.

As the nurses wheeled the gurney to the entrance, I couldn't see what was happening. I could see an exceptionally large woman overflowing from the gurney. From the little I could see, she was face-down and squirming. The nurse who pulled the front of the gurney was laughing so hard she had fat tears rolling down her cheeks. Our patient was screaming, and her husband was still in panic.

"Please," he begged the nurses, "don't let her die."

"Can't you go any faster?" the patient screamed. "I pay your salary with my taxes!"

Throughout her ten-second passing through the lobby and into the ER, the patient cursed, insulted, and belittled the nurses. I still couldn't see what was going on.

"Sir," one of the accompanying security guards said to the patient's husband, "you step up to one of these windows and register your wife."

The man argued and refused. Security had to explain four times that registering the patient was not only for our protection, but also hers. Finally, the man came to the window.

My window.

I took the patient's identifying information.

"And can you please tell me her complaint?" I asked.

The man shook his head. "Skip that part."

"Sir," I explained gently, "my screen won't let me skip that. I have to select something before I can finish the registration process."

He leaned in and was so close to the window that his breath fogged the glass. "She has a zucchini stuck in her…"

He pointed downward.

I selected 'foreign body in vagina' before allowing the man back to see his wife.

Shortly after this, one of the doctors called my line and yelled, "Why did you enter that complaint?"

I stammered and told him what the patient's husband just told me.

"It's not in her vagina," screamed the doctor. "You really need to get these things right. Change it."

I made the change on the patient's chart and my coworkers laughed. One said to me, "After you've been here a while, you'll learn to ask which hole it's in."

I nodded.

A nurse came to the desk, laughing her butt off.

"Anyone got a vegetable peeler?" she asked, before calling a patient from the waiting room.

We learned the 'zucchini' stuck in the patient's rectum was actually a large cucumber. The patient and her husband were fooling around in the bedroom and got a little carried away.

One of the nurses told us the patient experienced rectal prolapse and had to go to surgery, where a mesh sling was inserted. From what I understand, this is rare condition in relation to sexual experimentation.

I never saw the patient or her husband again, but I did hear that she was much nicer to the nurses on the surgical floor.

I didn't need more time to learn to ask patients 'which hole?' I learned that from this experience.

--H.T.

California

<u>Need Assistance Right Meow</u>

I answered a call from an excited elderly woman. She stated there was a 'rather large cat' stuck in a tree in her backyard. She told me she could not go to bed, knowing the cat was stuck, and she did not who else to call, so she called our fire house.

I joked with my partner and asked if he wanted to go on the call with me, so we hit the road in our maintenance F150, wearing only our civilian clothes.

We drove to the outskirts of our rural town until we pulled up at a nice brick ranch. An elderly woman peeked out from her front window and motioned for us to continue up her walkway. My partner continued around the caller's house, carrying a ladder. It was almost sundown and we wanted to release the cat and get back to the station.

The little old woman inside cracked her front door and asked, "Where's your gun?"

"I'm with the Fire Department, ma'am," I replied. "I don't carry a gun."

She shook her head and replied, "Oh, my. I think I called the wrong department."

As soon as she closed the door in my face, I stood on her stoop and kind of scratched my head. I began to wonder if the caller was senile or possibly just confused.

I heard my partner scream and the ladder clatter from the backyard and as I was jogging back there, my partner was sprinting out like he was competing in the Olympics. I saw the ladder on the ground next to a thirty-foot sycamore.

He yelled to me to run, and I didn't even know what I was running from, but I've seen enough scary movies to know that if someone yells that at me, I should probably just do it.

So, here you have two mildly out-of-shape men in their forties, who thought they were going to simply pull a tabby out of a tree before going back to the station for grilled brats and coleslaw, who are now running like a T-Rex was on the loose.

About halfway to the truck I looked over and asked my partner, "Why are we running?"

He panted, "It's not a cat."

I don't know what was going through my head at the time, but I can tell you I ran a lot faster once he told me that.

Once we were back in the truck and took a few minutes to catch our breaths, I asked my partner, "What was it?"

His eyes were as wide as pie pans when he told me, "It's a tiger. It's a damn tiger."

My partner had climbed the ladder and was face-to-face with the monster, who was ticked-off and took a swipe at him, which caused him to fall from the ladder.

We called over the radio for police assistance and explained our predicament.

The guys at the PD laughed and told us to stop screwing with them. It took ten minutes for them to take us seriously, and then it took another ten minutes for them to figure out what they were going to do and how a tiger ended up in the middle of South Dakota. We couldn't really call animal control to help us out because out here, we are animal control.

By the time the PD arrived on scene with their plan of 'shoot a net at it and then we'll go from there,' it was dark and the cat had yet another advantage over us weaklings on the ground. The animal was angry, growling loudly and menacingly fake-lunging at us. We were afraid it would either jump down or fall if the tree limbs broke, and then we'd all be in some hefty trouble.

After close to an hour of deliberation, we discovered the 'rather large cat' escaped from an exotic feline rescue center located two counties over. It had been missing for a full day, and none of us had any clue. We only found that out because we put out calls, looking for tranquilizer darts and someone certified to handle an animal of this caliber.

The owners of the rescue joined us. Our new plan was for all non-essential personnel to retreat to their vehicles. Two officers would remain in the yard as a backup plan, along with my partner and myself. One of the owners would shoot a tranquilizer dart at the cat, and if all went well, the animal would remain in the tree until it passed out and fell to an inflatable mat we set up at the tree's base. The owner told us to pray that the plan went well and hope the cat didn't pounce from the tree before the tranquilizer took effect, which was estimated between five and thirty seconds.

The problem with every part of that plan is this: when you're dealing with a 490-pound animal with no natural predators besides man, five-to-thirty seconds becomes a lifetime.

The cat's owner popped off the first tranq and missed. When the animal realized someone was shooting at him, he became further agitated and leapt. As he was coming down, the owner managed to pop off another tranq dart, which lodged in the center of the tiger's chest.

In a fit of rage, the cat went right for the officers on standby. The officers panicked (and rightfully so), and the cat went after the older of the two. We thought the cat was going for a swift kill, but he swatted the officer across the neck with his paw. Up until that night, I never recognized the power these animals possess. One easy swipe for the cat sliced the officer's neck, and once the cat smelled blood, he refused to back away from the officer. We called for the second officer to put the cat down, but she said she was afraid to move, even as blood was gushing from her partner's wounds.

Luckily, within a matter of seconds, the tranquilizer took effect and the cat passed out.

The injured officer was transported to the local hospital for sutures. He said he'd rather have the stitches than a toe tag, and we couldn't agree more. The tiger was transported to its rescue center and was then transferred to an open-roam facility that was better equipped to meet its needs to wander.

--M.Y.

South Dakota

Desperate Times, Desperate Measures

I was a medic for 32 years and have varied responses to the 'What was the worst thing you've seen?' question. We see so much out there that 1.) we don't want to relive it with someone who's just asking to get a rush, and 2.) 'worst' is subjective. For me, the worst of the worst calls always involved children. One of my partners didn't deal with elderly calls well. What's the 'worst' for you isn't going to be for someone else. I'm not sure I could put any one call in the 'worst' spot because every call regarding a drowned toddler or an infant who has choked on a button can fill the position. In the end, they all come back to haunt you.

Without a doubt, however, I can recall my most *disturbing* run.

It was back in 1999, when the Y2K stuff was hitting the fan. If you don't remember when this happened, people all over the world feared that our computers wouldn't be able to roll over to 2000, and to them, that meant power grids would fail, nuclear plants would explode, and satellites would fall from the sky. Many people lived their day to day lives with a ping of fear, the 'what if?' fear in the back of their minds, but some were downright crazy with this notion that the world was coming to an end.

On New Year's Eve, my partner and I were dispatched to a trauma in a local trailer park. We were all too familiar with the place. It was a scummy part of town, and I don't think a single decent person lived there. Some of the trailers had windows and front doors missing. Stray cats ruled the place, so you knew you were getting close when you could smell cat urine and drug residue. Most of the time, we requested police assistance, but the cops were out busting parties and taking care of traffic accidents, and at the time we placed our call, we were told we were S.O.L (crap out of luck), so we went alone.

We drove through crowds shooting off fireworks and handguns until we reached the second to last trailer at the end of this park. Our presence gathered the attention of everyone we passed, so the bus was surrounded by onlookers as soon as we stepped out. A small crowd had already gathered around the decrepit trailer.

As I grabbed my bag, a man ran from the trailer, fell off the four-foot-high deck, and smacked his nose against the ground. We helped him up and saw his nose was bleeding, busted from the impact. But this man was also soaked in blood, from his tank top, down to his socks.

My partner asked the man what happened, and his response was, "The Secret Service is after us because we bought shoes made in China."

I pulled my partner inside and told him to get back in the bus and demand police assistance. I then told him to meet me inside as soon as he finished, and to yell for me if he needed help.

As I pulled myself up on the deck with no stairs, I could already smell the meth residue from the trailer. I reached for a light switch and roaches the size of a Mack truck scurried down my fingers. I shook them off and realized there was no power to the mobile home.

I heard a man moan from the back room, and guiding myself in the dark with a flashlight, I waded through piles of junk mail and bugs, dirty and broken dishes, trash, feces, cats, and a few rats half the size of the cats. There wasn't much else in the trailer, but I could tell people lived there because there were clothes all over, draped over the few items of furniture there were. I passed a room that had a queen mattress on the floor, and then a bathroom that smelled like death.

In the back bedroom, I found a man in his late-20s. He was lying on the floor in a pool of blood, barely conscious, probably wishing he wasn't. His left ankle, just above an electronic monitoring device, was approximately 80-percent severed. I placed the flashlight in between my teeth and frantically tore through my bag, looking for anything that could help me.

As I crawled around on the dirty floor, kicking used needles out of my way, I accidentally dropped the flashlight. It rolled near the patient's head. Still in a crawl, I reached for the light. As I picked it up from the ground, I saw I was not alone with the patient.

The sliver of light illuminated the face of another man. He was also covered in blood, much of it splattered on his skin, and he was grinning as he stared into my eyes. He didn't say a word. I scanned the light downward.

The man was holding a bloodied hatchet.

I bolted from the trailer, scaring several of the cats in the process. As soon as I hit the front deck, I tripped over one of the strays and fell off the porch, landing on my back. My partner exited the bus and came to check on me. He told me a police escort was on the way.

I pulled him aside again and explained the situation. We agreed that neither of us would enter the trailer until the police arrived. Many of the onlookers had disappeared back to their drugs and alcohol, and I scanned the dark park.

"Where's that first guy?" I asked.

My partner shrugged. "I saw him walk off. Figured he'd come back."

Two patrol cars arrived on scene and a set of officers entered the trailer, with weapons drawn. We heard a lot of yelling, but they returned with the hatchet-wielder in cuffs. They made him sit in the yard.

Our audience was back.

The officers set up yellow tape around the trailer's perimeter and instructed bystanders to leave the scene. My partner and I entered the trailer, but by this point, our patient had expired from blood loss. The coroner later concluded that the man would have died regardless, as we arrived on scene far too late to keep him alive.

After the hatchet-wielder came down from his high and the first busted-nose man was found a few trailers away, we learned the men were high on PCP when they thought the patient's ankle monitor was a tracking device placed by the government. They believed the Secret Service wanted to kill them, so when they couldn't cut the device from the man's ankle, they decided to chop off his limb.

I did not take leave following the incident, but I should have. I started having anxiety attacks when we were called to other trailers, to the point that my boss ordered me to go to counseling and I was prescribed medication. To this day, I can't watch horror movies where ghosts or ghouls are lingering in a dark corner, and this happened more than a decade ago. I still have nightmares every now and then.

--R.E.

Florida

Dog Nabbit

I was a tech in a busy ER and one night, I couldn't catch a break for the life of me. Nurses were shouting constant orders for me to do something, and before I could finish, they had already shouted eighty more things to do.

I entered a room, stripped the bedding, and replaced it. I knew for a fact that I did it, so when a nurse demanded to know why 'her' room didn't have a blanket, I didn't know what to tell her. I explained until my face was blue that I knew I placed a blanket on the bed, and there was nothing she could say that would convince me otherwise. I had been doing the job for two years at that point, so I knew what I was doing.

To satisfy the nurse's demands, I took a fresh blanket from our warmer and placed it over the bed's thin sheet. I positioned the single standard-size pillow at the head of the bed. Then, I turned off the lights as I left the room.

A few minutes later, the same nurse confronted me in the hall as I was holding a bedpan. She belittled me in front of my peers and patients, and she demanded to know why I replaced the blanket but took the pillow from the room. It was starting to feel like I was on one of those prank shows.

I informed the nurse that I did not remove the pillow from the room, but the nurse did not believe me. She yelled at me, called me stupid, and said that I was purposefully trying to make her angry. Someone bumped me from behind and I fell forward. The contents of the bedpan splashed on the nurse's scrubs. She called me more names and told me to have the room finished by the time she returned from changing her scrubs.

Frustrated, I entered the room a third time. I replaced the missing pillow, and then I left the room again. I stood at the end of the hall, hoping to catch the person responsible for removing the previous items. A patient on the other side of the room coded and I was called to assist with machinery.

When I was released from my duty with that room, I was confronted again. The nurse walked me to the room, screaming the entire way, and told me she was writing me up because now the pillow *and* the blanket were gone.

I was so angry that I began to cry. I told the nurse that if she wanted to write me up, she could do it. I knew I had done my job properly, and I wasn't about to let someone tell me I hadn't.

As I was leaving the room, a large golden dog with a fat belly and matted fur peeked in the room and ran back the automatic doors that opened to our dumpster area. I followed the dog outside and saw two blankets and two pillows piled behind the airflow unit. I went back inside and made the nurse wait with me. We watched the dog sneak back inside the ER, enter the room, and scurry back outside while dragging another blanket behind her.

I thought seeing that would make the nurse apologize to me, but she never did. Instead, she ordered me to call someone to remove the dog from hospital grounds, and she made me scrub the entire room and hall where the dog had walked.

I quit the next day and cited the nurse's behavior as my reason.

The thief dog was taken to the shelter and she was found to be pregnant. I adopted one of her puppies when they were ready to for homes.

--J.O.

Illinois

At a fertility consultation, we got down to the root of the problem as to why a couple could not conceive.

After never-ending questions, we discovered the wife was still taking her birth control pills because, while she was still wishing to conceive, she wanted to regulate her painful and irregular periods.

--B.L.

West Virginia

Kitten a Little Crazy in Here

I'm a head nurse in our ER and I am convinced our local police department hates us. I say that jokingly, but there are times I wonder.

Intake called me to the front because a male patient in his late teens was in the lobby, curled up on the floor and sobbing. The clerk could not register the patient and did not know what to do.

I approached the young man and asked him to describe his problem. He cried, "I called the cops and they told me to come here."

I asked the young man again to tell me what was wrong. He stated he visited a friend's drug dealer to purchase marijuana. He had never smoked before but wanted to try it. However, after smoking an entire joint, his friend informed the patient that he did not smoke marijuana. The dealer gave the patient a joint filled with catnip.

The young man repeated to me that he did not want to die. He wanted us to "pump [his] stomach or something."

I was close to tears as I attempted to convince the young man to stand up. I had to stifle my laughter, which made me cough, and before I knew it, I could hardly breathe from choking on air.

An officer arrived while I was laughing. He asked, "Catnip boy?"

I nodded and the patient screamed, "Oh my God, everyone knows I'm dying and that's what they're going to call me when I'm gone."

I was laughing so hard at that point that I wanted to lie down on the floor, too.

After several minutes of this, we registered the patient and informed him that he was in the clear. An officer gave the teen a lecture on drug usage and the teenager willingly disclosed the dealer's address and identity.

The dealer was arrested for possession and distribution of cannabis. I guess he told the cops that he did not trust our patient, so he gave the teen catnip instead of weed.

We discharged our patient and told him to stay off the drugs…and the nip.

--P.Y.

Oregon

<u>Jump</u>

I have been employed by a fantastic department for several years now, and I love my job. About three years ago, I ended an average shift and came home to my fifth-floor apartment. It's not much, but it's just me, so I don't need a lot of space.

Because my apartment is small, it wasn't difficult to pick up on the scent of stale cigar smoke and beer. I neither smoke nor drink, so I knew right off the bat that someone had been in my apartment. My front door had been locked, meaning the only entrance for an intruder was the balcony door, which I had left open to bring in fresh air.

I placed my hand on my weapon and turned to enter my bedroom. I searched the room and closet before moving to the bathroom. Nobody was in there, either. As I was approaching the kitchen, a man darted across the apartment, ran through the sliding screen door, and leapt from the balcony, taking the mesh screen with him. Outside, people screamed.

I don't know if I was more startled at seeing someone in my apartment or fearing that I was about to have to call in a dead body.

Much to my surprise, as soon as I stepped out on the balcony, I saw the man from my apartment pick himself up from the ground and run. Mind you, he just jumped from a fifth-floor apartment so he wasn't in tip-top shape, but he retained his ability to flee.

I put in a call for residential entry and beach patrol found the guy a few miles down. He was found climbing balconies and checking doors.

You would think that, as an officer, I would have known better than to leave my glass door open, but I honestly never thought some fool would climb up five floors in broad daylight. I saw absolutely no harm in airing out my apartment and never in a million years thought someone would do something like that.

I use this story to remind everyone to remain vigilant and never think it won't happen to you.

--M.U.

Florida

<u>Happy Halloween</u>

Nobody ever believes this story, but here it is.

The morning after Halloween, a man and woman stepped up to my registration booth and said they both wanted to be seen by mental health. I gave both a clipboard with paperwork to fill out and instructed them to return everything to me when they were finished.

Though the woman took her paperwork to the waiting area, the man informed me he could not complete the forms.

"Sir, your girlfriend can complete them for you, if you'd like, but I really must insist they're completed," I said to him.

Without warning, the man vomited on the floor. It reeked of alcohol. He pleaded to be seen immediately and would not move from the registration area.

Nobody else was around because it was still dark outside, so I registered the man as I would for an ambulance patient, and then I pressed the button that notified triage of a new patient. The man thanked me and started to cry. He vomited three more times into an emesis bag.

The man's girlfriend came to the desk and sheepishly handed me her paperwork. She asked how long it would take to be seen, and I informed her it would not be too long. She sniffled and returned to the waiting room.

While the girlfriend was waiting for triage, she too vomited. I thought maybe the two had gone on a bad binge the night before. I was surprised college kids weren't coming in, but I figured half were in jail from being clearances the night before, while the others were still asleep. It was going to be a long day of vomiting and hangover complaints.

Triage called the girlfriend and they went to a room.

About ten minutes later, the triage nurse came sprinting to the counter like someone had set the back room on fire. She was jumping up and down and had her hands clamped over her mouth.

"What are you doing?" I asked her. "What happened?"

"That wasn't his girlfriend," she laughed loudly.

I shrugged and said, "Oh, my bad."

She was holding her breath and trying not to laugh, and she was so red and swollen that she looked like she was going to burst at the seams.

"What?" I asked.

The triage nurse explained our patients attended a Halloween party and had consumed copious amounts of alcohol before they ended up in bed with each other, a random hookup for both. When they woke up, they became ill and drove to the hospital.

I could not understand why this was so funny, but then the nurse explained, "They're brother and sister."

Now, I know this sounds like a cheesy, raunchy urban legend, but I swear everything about it is true. The woman was discharged, but the man was admitted for observation because he threatened to kill himself.

--K.L.

Indiana

Security once detained a man for trying to steal a TV from our ER waiting room. This man just walked in, stood on a chair, unplugged the TV, and then lifted it off its brackets and tried to walk out the door like he just bought the thing at a yard sale.

It was the weirdest thing I've encountered at work. I still wonder if he really thought he could get away with it.

--T.M.

New Jersey

Use the Force…It's Logical

I work in registration in our ED and last Halloween was terrible. Now, before I start, *every* Halloween around here is terrible because we have three colleges in our city. Every year, we see slutty versions of every costume you could imagine. We deal with ETOH kids all year long, but on Halloween we schedule additional staff to the ED. Every year, it's like this.

During the last Halloween shift, we were just as busy as I thought we'd be. A slutty cat arrived with a slutty bunny and a slutty version of the least-slutty cartoon ever: Maggie Simpson. Kitty had been fighting with Maggie but the two had since made up. They were both puking. Bunny probably had no business driving, but Kitty needed stitches after being hit in the forehead with a broken beer bottle.

We saw two Power Rangers and one Teenage Mutant Ninja Turtle for an MVA, and then we signed in a guy dressed as a Christmas tree for mental health.

For four hours, it was like this. I considered stabbing myself with scissors just so I could clock out and go home, but my coworker reminded me that in order to make it deep enough to leave, I'd probably have to cut deep enough to also get stitches. And, well, since the ED was full, it wasn't worth it. I'd rather sit at my counter than become a patient and have to sit in the waiting room with Snow White barfing on the floor and Wreck-It Ralph trying to get me in bed. I couldn't even take my lunch break because Halloween nights are so busy we all clock out 'no lunch,' and I had forgotten my snacks at home, so I had to just sit there and suck it up. Only eight more hours to go.

Close to midnight, our Star Wars characters came in. We had the classics: Darth Vader, Luke Skywalker, Leia (in the slave costume, what else?), and Chewbacca. I found Chewbacca to be the funniest in the group, only because in the movies Chewy was tall, but the version in our lobby was on someone who was maybe just over five-feet.

Darth Vader came to the desk, but we couldn't understand the guy over the sound of his mask. The mask had a battery-operated sound effect built in, so every few seconds it sounded like he was huffing paint.

Leia came to the desk and was a royal pain in the butt. This girl apparently thought she was royalty, too. She demanded to go see her friend, who hadn't even arrived via ambulance yet. Leia informed us several partygoers had gotten sick from spiked punch at a frat party, so we were going to receive approximately 20 more barfing, drunk, stupid, and belligerent patients. How fun!

We sent the Star Wars group to the waiting area, where Darth and Chewy started greeting the Hulk and a pregnant nun. Luke was busy using his plastic lightsaber to lift the skirt of a slutty ballerina, and Leia was yelling at him because he was 'being a perv.'

The next group we saw walk in were dressed as characters from Star Trek. In front of me stood Captain Kirk, Spock, an unnamed

Red Shirt, and...Worf. Worf stated he liked Star Trek: The Next Generation better than the original series. I guess he picked up on the look I was shooting at him.

Our Trekkies were also there to visit friends from the frat party. We told them to go to the waiting room, and everyone but the Red Shirt complied. One of the security guards told the guy that if he couldn't listen to simple instructions, he'd be walked off premises and he'd be the first to go from his group, just like on the show. His friends laughed and they all went to the waiting room.

As expected, tons of college kids showed up for their friends. Ambulances were coming in left and right. We were setting ED patients up in our Rehab ward down the hall. At one point, we ran out of emesis bags and someone had to send security to raid a local clinic. The guards came back with three huge boxes and saved the day.

While we were registering Little Bo Peep for an ankle injury, I heard shouting from the waiting room and glanced over. Kirk and Luke were chest-to-chest, screaming in each others' faces about which cult had the better story line and characters. Spock and Chewy got involved. Before I could call security out to settle them down, Chewy took off his mask and clocked Worf. Chewbacca turned out to be a woman. Worf said he wouldn't hit a woman, but he would hit a man, so in return, he punched Luke.

The fight was on.

What began as Star Wars versus Star Trek became an all-out brawl between the fifty-something college kids in the waiting room. My coworker called security and told me to call the police, which I did immediately.

Our security department sent all available guards to the waiting room, but they only had one man and one woman available. The female guard was having better luck because none of the men would hit her. Then, someone changed that, so our female guard was on the floor with a bloody nose. Part of the group turned from the original fight and started beating the crap out of the guy who hit the female guard. Our male guard used his stun gun on two people but became overwhelmed by attacks, so he helped the other guard up and they were registered to be seen for their injuries.

Once the police arrived, it was a sight to be seen. All these movie, television, and comic book characters were racing in all directions, trying to find exits or places to hide. There was still a massive fight taking place in the center of the waiting room, but the participants had dwindled from fifty-something to maybe a dozen. Officers gave the group three chances to lie down on the ground, but only one person did. The rest were shot with bean bags, and two people were pepper sprayed.

Out of the group, I'd say we had close to 20 additional patients register for injuries, just from the fight.

To make that entire situation worse, I had to go to rooms to talk to patients and the Yoda from the Star Wars group was drunk and only spoke in backwards language.

In the course of 12 hours, I think we saw more than 200 patients, and a good 90-percent of them were imbecile college kids.

Honestly, that night was maybe my worst night of work in all the years I've worked at this hospital. I can't wait to finish my teaching program and peace-out of this place.

--D.G.

Louisiana

Grateful to Be Alive

Dispatch sent me to respond to a report of a male in his 60s-70s, seizing in a car that had been swerving erratically on the interstate. The male pulled to the side of the road and was thought to continue seizing.

When I pulled behind his vehicle, I could see his head bobbing back and forth, from side to side, and he occasionally smacked his head against his seat's headrest.

I approached the man's vehicle and noticed his car windows were rattling.

It took three taps on the man's driver's side window before he noticed I was at his door. He jumped, turned down his radio, and cracked the window.

"Sir," I said, "concerned motorists called 911 because they believed you were having seizures while driving. We had reports that you were driving erratically. EMS is on the way."

The man seemed confused for a moment, but then he laughed.

"I wasn't having no seizure," he told me. "My daughter just bought me the Grateful Dead's greatest hits."

The man explained how the music 'took him back,' and he had been dancing. He decided to pull over when he almost hit a semi-trailer.

I called in a disregard to EMS and listened to a few songs with the man before I told him to keep the dancing to a minimum while he was driving.

--N.A.

Arizona

Superhero

The worst call of my life happened in the mid-80s, when my partner and I were dispatched to a home on the other side suburbia. We were responding to a 911 call made by a panicked neighbor. All we knew was that a child was burned. We didn't know how, the child's age, or the child's condition. Dispatch warned us that the child's mother could be heard screaming frantically in the background of the phone call.

When we arrived on scene, we saw no indication of a fire from the home's drive. The home was located in a nice subdivision, the kind with grass so green you think you're in heaven. You know the place; nothing bad could ever possibly happen here.

As we moved up the walkway, we could hear a woman shrieking and begging for help. Just as we were about to knock on the door, it flew open and a woman in her mid-50s motioned us to upstairs. She was crying and kept saying, "It's bad. It's really bad."

We moved through the immaculate home until we reached the upstairs bathroom.

My partner immediately turned away and vomited on the hall carpet.

I stood there for maybe half a second, but it felt like two years. On the tile floor laid a child no older than seven. Blood and plasma pooled around him, mixed with puddles of water and sludge. His mother knelt over him and scrubbed at his skin with a wet washcloth, and as she did, his skin peeled. The room smelled like a mixture of sulfur, burnt hair, bleach, and ammonia. Liquid in the tub gave off what appeared to be steam, as the bath of chemicals interacted with each other.

"I was just doing yard work," his mother screamed. "Help him. Please, help him."

I ran inside the bathroom and tripped on empty bottles of bleach, acidic clog remover that I had seen packaged at stores in industrial-strength plastic casing, bathroom cleaners, and a box of borax. It looked as if he'd taken every cleaner he could find and poured it in the bathtub.

The child was nude. His clothes were in a messy pile between the tub and toilet, where a comic book rested on the closed toilet seat.

My chest felt tight as I attempted to assess the child's chemical burns. My stomach ached. The gas buildup in the bathroom was becoming toxic. We had to move the unresponsive child and his family out of the bathroom and soon, but I had no idea how to go about moving him.

I pressed my latex glove to the child's throat to feel for a pulse. A chunk of his thin skin stuck to my fingers like packing tape. As I lifted his arm, skin stuck to the tile floor and ripped from his body. If we moved him, his posterior would peel. If we left him, he would die, either from the burns, the shock, or the fumes.

The child's mother babbled. "All he's been talking about this week is getting superpowers." The rest was incoherent.

My partner was still in the hall, with his back turned to the scene. She said she couldn't come inside. I explained to the child's mother and neighbor that we had to move everyone out of the room. I also explained the possibility of the child's skin adhering to the tile floor and separating from his body. His mother argued at first, but then she screamed to save him at any cost.

When I lifted the child in my arms, I could feel his flesh against my arms and the chemicals leaking from his body singed my own skin. I called for my partner to assist, but she vomited again.

I positioned the child in the back of the truck and asked my partner to drive. I think that's the shortest and longest trip in the history of transport. The entire time, the child's mother cried over his limp body. He was breathing, but barely. When I bagged him, the skin around his mouth and nose crumpled and ruffled under the suction. I had to stop, in fear of further injuring him. There was absolutely nothing we could do for him, except get him to the hospital.

Once we arrived to ES, there was an argument between the doctors, nurses, and the patient's mother. Protocol stated all chemical exposures were to enter decon prior to being placed in a room. At the same time, with the extent of the child's degloving, we did not know if it was the right route to go. Pediatrics and surgeons were stat paged, including those off duty. Everyone scrambled to help the child, but none of us knew what to do.

In an executive decision, one of the doctors rolled the child to the decon room and turned the showers on. He called for nurses to assist. My partner was crying in the hallway and talking about her own son, who'd just turned five. Undoubtedly, it was the most difficult call for her at the time as well.

In the decon room, as the patient was exposed to water, his condition worsened and he stopped breathing. Unfortunately, there was nothing doctors could do for the child. His autopsy found chemicals in his stomach and lungs, bringing us to the theory that the child had submerged himself in the chemicals for some time, before the burning set in. The coroner also found a fresh gash on the child's head, suggesting the boy attempted to get out of the tub but fell in. This fit with the mother's testimony that the child was unresponsive at the time she found him in the bathtub.

My partner quit when we arrived at the station. She said she signed up to help people and failed, and that she could not chance risking someone's life if she should ever have the same reaction in the future.

I now have children of my own and can tell you that when they were younger, none of them were allowed in the bathroom unattended, even to use the restroom, due to my fears of this happening to them. My wife never could understand. I still haven't told her about this call because I don't think she could handle it. It was the worst thing I've ever seen in my entire life.

--Initials and location withheld at request

Skate on By

I was dispatched to the abandoned high school in our rural community, due to a noise complaint. I've been on the force for several years, and this is nothing unusual for our aging community. Folks hardly leave this area. When they do, they come back to live in peace and quiet, so the majority of our calls revolve around loud mufflers, music, or kids out being kids.

When I arrived, it was dusk. I took a flashlight and went through most of the first and second floor of the building. I didn't hear or hear much. Someone had busted out a few windows, so I would occasionally cross paths with a racoon or cat.

As I was preparing to exit the building, I heard crying from the first-floor gymnasium. When I attempted to open the double doors, I could not. I knocked on the doors a few times, thinking the person(s) inside had barricaded themselves in the gym, but I heard the typical shushes from inside the room.

I was mighty frustrated at this point because it was dark and there are no working streetlights surrounding the building, nor is there power in the facility. We were due for a nasty storm that was forecast to start at any minute, and I was supposed to be off duty a half hour earlier, with the entire weekend off.

I walked around the building, until I reached the back part of the gymnasium. There was a small ladder leading up to a series of broken windows. What was most peculiar about this scene, however, is that there was also a garden hose snaked through the window. I visually traced the hose—which was connected to at least three other hoses—back to the trailer park.

Hand to God, I won't lie; I cursed up a storm as I climbed the ladder and peeked inside. At first, as I attempted to scan the room with my light, I couldn't see much. I could hear a couple of kids somewhere in the room. One was crying and the other whispered, "Shut up."

I couldn't see jack with my flashlight without getting closer, so I leaned in the gymnasium and told the trespassers that I would only give them a warning if they came out of hiding.

"We can't," said a boy. "He's hurt."

Oh, Jiminy Christmas.

I pushed myself through that window and landed flat on my keister, and it wasn't because of the way I landed. My landing was fine. Both soles of my boots hit the surface flat.

But the surface was made of ice.

I scanned the floor.

The entire gymnasium floor was covered in what I would estimate to be four-inches of ice.

It was a trial to move across the room to get to two teenagers. I know the boys quite well, so I am not the least bit surprised that they used their garden hose to flood the gym in intervals, allowing the floor to ice over before adding another layer of water.

Both teens were wearing shoddy ice skates when I reached them. One teenager had fallen while goofing around and broke his ankle and wrist. His friend said the boys were too afraid to go for help. I don't know what the dingalings were going to do overnight.

I radioed for a medical team and let them extract the boys from the building.

I decided against ticketing the kids. The fact that one fell and broke bones was a good enough punishment, and the building was set for demolition in Spring, anyway.

I never told them, but I am mighty impressed with their ingenious plan.

--K.A.

Kentucky

<u>Relax</u>

I work at a well-known health store as a pharmacist. One evening, I noticed a young man seemed to be having difficulties finding a product, so I stepped out to assist him.

"Do you need help finding something?" I asked.

He nodded and said, "I'm looking for those pills that help you relax, like that chick took in that Sixteen Candles movie."

"Muscle relaxers?"

"Yeah!" he exclaimed.

"Those can be pretty powerful," I cautioned. "Are you sure you don't just need aspirin or ibuprofen?"

He shook his head and said, "Oh, it's for someone else. She has extreme tightness."

I shrugged and helped the man select a bottle of OTC muscle relaxers. We reviewed the dosage information on the back, as well as potential side effects. The man paid, took the pills, and left the store.

Probably about an hour, maybe hour-and-a-half after he left, I received a call. It was the same man.

"I have a question about those pills," he told me.

"Let me see if I can help," I said.

"Well, they're supposed to relax muscles, right?"

"That's right. Did the person take the correct dosage?"

"I think so," the man answered. "But see, we're trying anal for the first time, and it's still really hard to get in there, man. Like, she's not any more relaxed than before she took these pills."

I laughed and told the man to try using more lubricant.

The young man came back in soon after the phone call and asked me to help him select that, too.

That's surely not the strangest customer experience I've ever had, but it is one of the most memorable.

--J.B.

Wisconsin

<u>Delivery</u>

Food delivery…yeeesh. After visiting hours, delivery men and women have to stop at the ER information desk. We have to page the employee or family expecting the food, and we have to buzz them back through the building. Sometimes we have two deliveries, but other nights we see the same delivery person so many times that they should just get a room.

In our department, the nurses get together and order food as a group. Then, they take a collection for a tip. Everyone in town knows that when you order from our department, you're going to walk out with at least a thirty-dollar tip. I've seen delivery people leave with a hundred bucks before. It just depends on the kind of night we're having or what bills we have to chip in.

One night, we ordered from a local pizza joint. Two delivery women showed up with more than ten pizzas, breadsticks, pasta, drinks—you get it; we ordered a bunch of food. We invited other departments to eat with us, so the delivery women split a tip $200 tip. They both seemed pleased when they left.

Someone forgot to move a nurse's plain cheese pizza from the rest of the food, and it was eaten. She has allergies and couldn't eat the other food, so she ordered another cheese pizza for herself. She gave me a twenty and asked me to pay the delivery person when he or she arrived. The total was something like $18, so she said to give the change to the driver as a tip. Since we just spent so much money on our order and a tip, I didn't think that sounded unfair.

The delivery person for the nurse's pizza was one of the women from the previous delivery. We completed the transaction, but when I told her the nurse said to keep the change as a tip, the woman became irate and refused to hand me the pizza. She said she wasn't going to leave until I called the nurse to the desk.

I called the nurse and she came up to the desk with a smile on her face, thankful that her food had arrived.

"What's with this crappy tip?" the delivery woman yelled.

The nurse and I tried to explain we felt the tip was fair, considering she had left just a half hour earlier with a hundred-dollar tip, not counting all the times she had delivered to other departments and families that night.

"So?" screamed the woman. "That was then. This is now. You think this two dollars means anything to me?"

The woman threw the nurse's tip to the floor and said she was not leaving until she received a proper tip.

Our nurse, beside herself at this point, told the delivery woman to take the pizza back to the restaurant. She told the delivery woman that she would be calling the restaurant to report her behavior.

No sooner than the words escaped the nurse's mouth, the delivery woman opened the pizza box and shoved the steaming pizza in our nurse's face. I called 911 and yelled for help while the phone was ringing.

An orderly and janitor pulled the pizza delivery woman off our nurse and we registered the nurse as a trauma. She sustained first and second degree burns to her face and had to take time from work.

The delivery woman was arrested for assault and was fired. I think the nurse sued her, but I don't know what happened with that in the end.

That incident convinced administrators to hire security.

--L.N.

Connecticut

<u>Squeaky Clean</u>

I responded to a call of a man passed out in a laundromat. What dispatch neglected to tell me is that the man was *inside* a washing machine, from the waist down. When I woke him up, he said he had been drinking and had explosive diarrhea. He reasoned a dollar for a wash cycle was cheaper than purchasing a change of clothes.

Jail clearance BAC was .35.

He still seemed proud of his decision when he woke up in our drunk tank.

--T.R.

New York

Bully

I retired from nursing in a medical facility to work as a school nurse. I love my job and wanted to share this with you.

A legally blind third-grader and his service dog had been the victims of a bully year-long. School administrators did not want to punish the bully because he was a staff member's child. Knowing he would only get a slap on the wrist, the fellow third-grader continued bullying his classmate, and his behavior became worse as the year continued.

One day, when the teacher stepped out of the classroom, the bully moved to physically assault the blind boy. Taking matter in his own hands, the child's dog pulled away from his owner and cornered the bully. Classmates said the dog did not snarl or bite until the bully hit the dog with a yardstick.

The bully ended up in my office with a superficial bite to the forearm while we awaited an ambulance. To add insult to injury, he had peed his pants in front of twenty other children.

I thought administration would call for the service dog to be removed from the school setting, but after his family threatened to sue, all charges were dropped.

I'm happy to report the child and his dog are no longer bullied.

--K.K.

Rhode Island

<u>Homegrown</u>

I have been a nurse for 32 years and never have I witnessed something like this.

A female, in her 60s, with a history of mental health and alcohol abuse diagnoses and admissions, was transported to our facility via EMS. She complained of a headache, shortness of breath, dizziness, was tachycardic, had an active nasal bleed, and she experienced nausea. We attributed some of her symptoms to her unusually high blood pressure and moved to treat that first.

The patient's condition, despite rigorous treatment, was not improving. It felt like we were in an episode of *House* because we could not figure out what we were doing wrong. We needed to know what we were facing to properly treat the patient and bring her to full health.

Our physician instructed us to interview the patient, believing she had been exposed to an agent in her home. Eventually, through speaking with the patient's daughter, we learned the patient had been attempting to produce homemade penicillin. This was dually confusing to us because the patient did not have a condition that would warrant the use of penicillin. We assumed her mental state attributed to her belief that she needed it.

Extensive testing showed our patient was suffering from mycotoxin (aflatoxin) poisoning via consumption and airborne exposure. Her condition was worsened due to her alcohol dependence and other health issues.

After consulting several physicians, toxicologists, and research centers, the patient was moved to ICU. The treatment plan included patient isolation, as her immunity could be compromised as she was weaned off the toxins. Professionals administered antioxidants and vitamins in multiple daily sessions, an attempt to flush the toxins from the patient's system.

Unfortunately, because the patient's immune system weakened, she expired six days following admission. Medical officials suggested her daughter contact a cleanup crew to safely enter her mother's residence prior to allowing anyone else in the home.

--Initials and location withheld at request

I responded to the hospital for a collision complaint and the patient showed me the motorcycle he had just wrecked.

He was arrested, because two hours earlier I took the report of the vehicle being stolen.

Moral of the story: if you steal something, don't show it off to an officer.

--B.F.

Ohio

Fidget Spinner

We received two back-to-back GSWs on an already busy evening shift. When I went back to gather information from the victims, I learned they lived at the same address and had been shot at their residence. Neither victim would initially release information as to what transpired. From what we could see, a .45 bullet had entered a female's leg through and through, exited, and struck a male's leg. Both patients were in their thirties.

There is absolutely no way around notifying law enforcement in a GSW case, so we called the authorities. At the same time two officers arrived, a middle-aged male arrived and asked to visit the patients. Officers agreed the male could visit, as long as he remained quiet during questioning and while they took their reports. The male agreed to this and we escorted him to the patients.

After a short time, the officers came to the front to chat. They stated the patients both gave the same word-for-word story that a friend had accidentally discharged a weapon while cleaning it, but the officers believed the story was bogus.

While the officers were at the desk, we heard shouting from the treatment area. The officers went back to investigate the source of the commotion and lend assistance, if needed.

We learned the commotion came about when the male visitor blamed the female for him shooting her. After officers broke up the argument that had somehow moved to the corridor, all parties confessed that the female was in possession of a fidget spinner. The male visitor asked to play with the device, but the female refused. When she refused to share the device, the male drew a firearm. The female did not believe the male would shoot her, so she further refused to hand over the fidget spinner. Agitated, the male shot the female, and as previously stated, the bullet traveled through her leg and hit her boyfriend's leg.

Officers arrested the male visitor for illegal possession of a firearm and for several open warrants.

--H.A.

Indiana

Little Ears Hear

Back in the 90s, we received a patient who had been sustained severe burns to approximately 40-percent of her body. Her injuries were horrific, but the story behind them were downright scary. We knew this woman as a former CNA, and all this time later, we still can't believe it happened to her.

The patient met her husband about a year earlier. Her husband then had a three-year-old son of whom he and his ex-wife shared custody. Our patient had complained several times that the child's mother was 'psycho.' She said that the ex-wife would call the house nonstop, stalk her, and once attempted to assault her. Our patient said the ex-wife's behavior became so concerning that the patient acquired an order of protection against the ex.

When the ex-wife was restricted from directly harassing the patient, she began instructing her son to do things to instigate trouble. For example, the patient once came to work with a chunk of her hair missing and stated that her stepson had cut it off while she was sleeping. She said she asked the boy why he did it and he stated, "Mommy told me to."

The patient and her husband filed for sole custody of the child. In the meantime, the now four-year-old was still traveling between homes. His behavior had not improved, but the patient was determined not to lose her mind over this. Her and her husband's attorney was convinced the two would be granted sole custody, based on the ex-wife's behavior. Our patient was hanging on for dear life. She even quit her job to prove to the courts that the child would have a full-time care provider.

One night, while the patient was asleep and her husband was out of town on a business trip, her stepson entered the bedroom and used matches to light the patient's bedding on fire. He then lit her hair on fire. When the patient woke, she was in total panic. She attempted to put out the flames but couldn't. She sustained burns to her hands, face, legs, arms, and head. She still carried her stepson outside and passed out in the front yard. Her neighbors saw the house fire and called 911.

We later learned the child said that his mother said she wanted the stepmom to die and 'burn in hell,' and the little boy attempted to make his mother happy.

I know the child was immediately removed from his mother's custody and placed with his father. The patient did survive and underwent several skin graft procedures to repair burns to her hands and extremities. She's been forced to wear wigs since this occurred.

The story received a small blurb in the local paper, and the whole town came together to offer support to our patient, but since it happened, it kind of faded away.

--Initials and location withheld at request

I had to take my wife to the hospital because I pulled back the shower curtain while wearing a latex horse mask, and she fell and busted her head open on the faucet. She didn't talk to me for two days.

--K.U.

Washington, D.C.

Call 911

    I was on standby medic call for 45 more minutes, but I hadn't been called in during my entire shift, so I thought I was in the clear. My daughter's friend was having a birthday party and the child's parents were in desperate need of a clown, after the one they hired skipped town with their non-refundable deposit and half of his wages. I do side work with Shriners, so I already had the supplies lying around the house. I did up my face, popped on a bulbous red nose, stuck a water-squirting flower in the breast pocket of my neon green suit jacket, and prepared my vehicle. Now, I think it's fitting that I drive a Smart Car, because you expect to see a clown in a tiny car, right? I take advantage of this by filling the car with balloons, so that when I step out at a party, the balloons come with me. I think it's a fun little surprise to add for the kids.

As I was driving down the interstate, I witnessed the car in front of me veer suddenly to the left and then to the right. It hit a guardrail with such force that the railing broke and the car rolled three times down the hill of a cavernous ditch. It came to rest upside down and there was smoke coming from the undercarriage and engine block.

Without hesitation, I pulled over, hit my hazard lights, and rushed down to the scene, balloons static-clinging to my suit. I could hear a man crying out a woman's name.

I could not gain entrance to the vehicle from the passenger side. The door was crumpled in on itself and the window was cracked, but I didn't have anything on me to break it. The woman inside was unconscious and bleeding from the forehead and nose.

When I saw the driver, a male in his 40s, was conscious, I raced to his side and was able to open the door, though it took some muscle.

I assessed the patient and smelled gasoline and smoke. We heard crackling and determined the vehicle was on fire. I informed the gentleman that we had to move him out of and away from the vehicle. As I moved to unbuckle him, I accidentally squirted myself in the face with my prank flower and some of my makeup got in my mouth, so I turned my head and made a series of spitting sounds and motions because the stuff tastes horrible.

"I'm not going with you," the driver yelled. "Call someone who knows what they're doing."

"Sir," I explained, "your vehicle is on fire and your passenger is unconscious. We need to move you away from the vehicle."

The man argued with me incessantly and refused to cooperate. He finally screamed at me, "Call 911!"

In a fit of exasperation, I replied loudly, "I am 911!"

I was out of breath as I explained to the demanding driver the reasoning behind being dressed as a clown. He still wasn't buying it and tried to go back to the vehicle four times to find his cell phone. Not one person from the interstate stopped or called in the crash.

The fire we heard was now visible and nearing the fuel tank. Flames raged in the back seat and turned the car's interior into a pit of hell.

The passenger was still unconscious.

I tried furiously to remove the woman's seatbelt, but it twisted and there was absolutely nothing I could do to cut the belt.

"In my car," I yelled to the driver, who was lying on the ground and complaining that he needed 'real' help, "there's a blue bag. It's bright blue, you can't miss it. Go get that bag."

I'll never forget what the man asked me.

"How do I know this isn't some plot to kidnap me and my wife?"

It's probably hard to imagine a clown with a painted-on grin to stare at you with a dead-serious expression, but that's what I did. I told the man that I couldn't run with my oversized red shoes on, and how I needed a tool from inside the bag to cut his wife's seatbelt. The bottom back of her seat was already on fire. I had to extract her from the vehicle. There was no time to waste.

Though he did so with a limp, the driver ran up the hill and returned in a matter of seconds with my supply bag.

"You take this clown gig seriously, don't you?" the man asked, nodding up to my car and the balloons that were blowing down the interstate.

I shook my head and I used what my buddies and I call the 'letter opener' (our crew hardly uses the cutters, but we are required to carry them) to free the passenger from her belt. Supporting her head and neck, her husband and I dragged her from the vehicle and we moved to a safe distance. I called in the accident and dispatch said, "Well, you're still technically on call for another six minutes, so just stay there."

I ended up missing the birthday party I volunteered to perform at, but I wouldn't change it for the world.

The passenger was fine. She smacked her nose against the dash on impact and it knocked her out. Obviously, the car was totaled.

I changed out of my clown gear and went to the hospital to check in on the patients. The driver apologized for how he reacted at the scene, but I understand that in times of stress we say and do things we wouldn't normally do.

My coworkers never let me live down the day they rolled on scene with me dressed as a clown.

--A.K.

Oklahoma

My 96-year-old hospice patient requested refried beans, enchiladas, and tamales for dinner. He said he finally had someone to clean up the mess to follow, so he could enjoy his favorite foods in his final days.

--D.S.

Alabama

Stuffed

I was dispatched to a residential dispute on Thanksgiving Day. When I arrived, three men were fist-fighting in the living room, four women were doing the same in the hallway, an old woman was screaming from the kitchen for everyone to stop, and two large teenage girls were…wait for it…they were literally stuck in the threshold that divided the living room and kitchen.

I called for backup and while I waited for assistance, I attempted to stop the fighting. That did not go well. The men were somewhat easier to break up, but they returned to their altercation. When I attempted to break up the all-female fight, I was elbowed in the face. I did draw my weapon, but none of the people in the house seemed to mind. I didn't feel it was necessary to fire, especially with assistance en route.

Two additional patrol cars arrived, each with two officers. We worked to separate and cuff all subjects involved in the physical altercations. We thought we were being gentle on the subjects by seating them on the sectional couch that wrapped around the living room, but even in cuffs they argued. One woman leaned over and bit another woman on the breast. She took a chunk of flesh in her teeth and everything.

We began loading the subjects in our vehicles, loading male-female, as to cut down on further assaults during transport. It was determined that our bite victim would not require EMS transport; I would take her to the local hospital for medical clearance prior to booking her in our facility. We didn't bother asking why the fight started. Here's a little secret that's not-so-secret: we usually don't care what started the fight. We just want everyone to stop acting like jackwagons for one day, just so we can catch a break. Apparently, that's too much to ask.

Once the subjects were loaded in vehicles, the additional patrols returned to headquarters.

I approached the kitchen threshold, where the two teenage girls were lodged tightly.

"Can you move at all?" I questioned.

One girl rudely replied with curses, "If we could move, we wouldn't be stuck here, stupid."

I nodded and tried to assess the situation. Neither girl could move her arms, but that did not stop the two from running their mouths-at me and at each other. As their argument persisted, the girl on the right headbutted the girl on the left, and then we had one teenager bleeding from a busted lip.

The thought in my head at the time was, 'I don't get paid enough for this.'

I planted my feet and leaned in, pushing on the girl on the right. I am a 5'5" female and weigh roughly 140-pounds. Each teenager probably weighed double what I do, at least. No matter how hard I pushed, the girl didn't budge.

From the kitchen, an elderly woman scolded the two teenagers for being overweight and greedy. She said she called to the family that dinner was ready, and the two teenagers raced each other to the kitchen. When they became stuck, comments were made amongst the family, which resulted in the altercation my coworkers and I had broken up.

With two subjects still in the back of my vehicle, I requested fire assistance. I did not know what else I could possibly do. There was no way I could dislodge the teenagers, and quite frankly, I was over the drama.

Fire arrived and attempted to dislodge the girls. They also failed. Grandma suggested using margarine to release the hold the girls had on each other and the door frame, but that did not work. After thirty minutes of futile attempts to dislodge the teenagers, two men from fire resorted to removing the door frame, which allowed the girls to dislodge with only minor scrapes and bruises.

You would think, that after all of this, the remaining family would be thankful to be out of this mess, but no.

The teenagers began fist fighting and their grandmother stood in the kitchen, screaming at them. I attempted to separate the teenagers, when one punched me. I used necessary force to bring her to her knees, and that's about the time the grandmother hit me with a ceramic coffee mug. Fire stepped in, we restrained the subjects, and I made yet another call for transport assistance.

Needless to say, the entire family spent Thanksgiving Day in jail.

--P.T.

Georgia

Eerie PD

I have received several 'ghost' stories from police officers. Here are a few:

■■■■■■■■■■■■■■■■■■■■■■■■■■■■■■■■■■■■■

I was on patrol one night and received a call from dispatch to respond to a complaint of young children playing on the train tracks near an abandoned trailer court. I did not know why kids would be out at three in the morning on a school night, but I responded just the same.

When I arrived, I could hear an approaching train in the distance, so I exited my vehicle and walked alongside the tracks, ensuring no children were in the train's path.

I walked an equivalent of half a block before I saw four children up ahead. They were laughing, calling out to each other, and appeared to be playing 'tag.'

I shined my light on one child and yelled, "Hey!"

Two of the children looked right at me but disregarded my presence. The railroad crossing arms lowered behind me, and the red flashing lights illuminated. The children were still on the tracks and showed no signs of moving.

I shouted for the kids to move off the tracks, but they still ignored me. At this point, I felt frightened at the idea that these kids were going to be hit by the train rumbling behind us.

In a panic, I ran toward the children, screaming like a madman the whole way. As I neared them, something strange happened.

All four children disappeared, right before my eyes.

I know I wasn't *that* tired. Obviously, someone else had either seen or heard the kids, too, so I couldn't have been imagining that they were there. I still have no idea what happened, but the only explanation I have is that they were never physically there in the first place.

I never told anyone what happened because I didn't want to hear that I was going crazy. I reported back to dispatch that the tracks were clear.

--Initials and location withheld at request

■■■■■■■■■■■■■■■■■■■■■■■■■■■■■■■■■■■■■■■

A year before this took place, some of our guys responded to a domestic dispute. When they arrived on scene, shots were fired inside the residence. An alcoholic husband and father shot the family's pets, two children, and wife, before turning the gun on himself. It was a terrible day for our town.

One year to the date of this, we received multiple calls reporting gunshots heard from the residence. It was a nightmare. We sent two patrols to the residence around noon, but the officers found nothing. The home had been abandoned since the initial incident, and when officers entered the home, they found it vacant.

Still, we received more calls throughout the day. Officers responded three more times, each time reporting the home was vacant.

Believing this was a prank by neighbors, I parked my patrol in the home's driveway at 21:00, hoping to deter callers.

For the first few minutes, everything was fine. I was prepared to sit in my patrol all night, if that's what it took.

After twenty minutes of sitting in my vehicle, watching Netflix on my phone, I heard gunfire from inside the residence. I exited the vehicle and banged on the front door, with my weapon drawn. I used the realtor's keys to enter the home when the gunfire ceased.

When I entered the home, it was vacant. As I searched the last bedroom of the home, which belonged to the family's daughter, I heard a woman scream from the kitchen, followed by another gunshot.

I raced to the empty kitchen and stood in its center. As I looked around in fear, a single gunshot rang throughout the kitchen. My ears were ringing, just as if I had fired my own weapon.

I have absolutely no explanation as to what occurred that day, but after midnight, we received no further reports of gunfire and never have again.

--X.W.

Alabama

∎∎∎∎∎∎∎∎∎∎∎∎∎∎∎∎∎∎∎∎∎∎∎∎∎∎∎∎∎∎∎∎∎∎∎∎∎∎∎

I was in my personal vehicle, on the way home from a 16-hour shift, when I almost hit a pedestrian. She was wearing a black sweater and black leggings; if my headlights hadn't reflected off one of her rings, I would have never seen her.

I almost went off the road to avoid this woman, who appeared to be in her early-20s.

When I stepped out of my truck, I asked the woman why she was walking in the road at midnight. I noticed she was crying, so I asked if she was hurt. She replied that she wasn't hurt, but she had been in an accident and her car was in a ditch a few miles down the road.

I offered the woman a ride, and we drove three miles before we saw a two-door sports car flipped on its side. I informed my passenger that I would call in the wreck, and I'd make sure she got home. She thanked me and said she was going to wait by her car. She exited my vehicle.

As I was calling in the accident, I looked away for a matter of seconds, and when I looked back, there was no wreck. I asked dispatch to hold, and I exited my truck. I called out for the stranger, but there was no response.

Shaken, I returned home and told my wife about what had occurred. She's a big believer in the paranormal and suggested an accident had occurred in that location and what I had encountered was an 'echo,' which she explained as 'spirits' left behind to repeat a traumatic experience. I laughed at the idea, but inside, her explanation was better than any I had.

A week later, we received a call of an MVA off mile marker 12. I knew the location well because that is where I drove the young woman I nearly hit with my truck.

When I arrived on scene, I was greeted by the coroner.

The vehicle was a two-door sports car, flipped on its side.

I passed out when I saw the deceased victim was my passenger a week earlier.

My supervisor ordered me to have a mental eval, but I'm not crazy. I know what I saw that night, and I know the MVA victim was the same young woman I drove down the road. I just can't explain it.

--Initials and location withheld at request

When Mr. Smith was still alive, he called 911 for every little thing.

Someone was walking a dog down the sidewalk in front of his house? 911.

He heard a car horn? 911.

The TV Guide said M.A.S.H was supposed to be on, but instead there was a baseball game airing? 911.

Because Mr. Smith was 102-years-old, we simply reminded him with each call that 911 was for emergencies only. His calls were such a habit that we became worried if he didn't call us.

One day, we received word that Mr. Smith's granddaughter found him deceased in his home. He had fallen asleep in his recliner and appeared to have passed peacefully of natural causes.

Oddly enough, Mr. Smith's phone number continued to dial 911. When we answered, we only heard an open line. Every now and then we would hear static on the line, but no voice. We figured the calls were the result of a faulty line.

Mr. Smith's granddaughter disconnected the phone service, but the phone calls continued. We would often receive two or three phone calls from the residence per day, and sometimes we would receive as many as fifteen empty-air calls from his home. We contacted his family and requested that they agree to allow a technician to enter the home and perform and diagnostics test of the line. The technician found no abnormalities with the disconnected phone line and could not explain why we were still receiving 911 calls from a residence where there was not even a phone.

On July 4th, as soon as our local fireworks began, calls from Mr. Smith's residence skyrocketed. We were answering nearly ten calls per hour for three or four hours before our dispatch threatened to quit. Out of frustration, I went to Mr. Smith's house and entered the residence. I calmly explained to the open-air, vacated residence that the influx of 911 calls were causing distress to our staff, and they needed to stop.

After that, we never received another 911 call from Mr. Smith's residence.

It sounds strange, but I promise on my life that it's true. I hope Mr. Smith moved on to bigger and better things.

--W.G.

Delaware

■■■■■■■■■■■■■■■■■■■■■■■■■■■■■■■■■■■■■■■

Officers were contracted out as overnight security at an electronics warehouse while their security team went on strike for better wages and working conditions.

I was the only person in the building, as far as I knew, but the motion-activated alarms kept going off near an emergency exit. I checked the alarms and doors several times, but finally gave in and figured the alarms near that exit were faulty. I made a note for management to call the alarm company the next day and instead of investigating the alarms again, I simply sat in the control room and blindly pressed the silence button, all while catching up on movies I had downloaded.

My tablet started to die, so I set it down and moved to grab my charger from an adjacent desk. As I moved, I noticed on security monitors a man nearing the emergency exit. The alarms activated, and I rushed down to the location to finally bust the cause of all my night's distress.

When I arrived at the location, the emergency exit was still closed. I looked around and there wasn't a soul in sight.

Defeated, I decided to return to the control room. I started to think I was tired and imagining things.

As I turned to return to my movie, I stood face to face with a man who looked every bit as real as I was. He was wearing a blue dress shirt that was tucked into his navy slacks. He stared straight ahead, but it was as if he didn't see me.

I took a step back as the man approached, but he continued toward me until he passed *through* me. It felt like I had swallowed a bucket of ice and had been electrocuted at the same time.

I asked around and heard from a few guys at the warehouse that a guy had committed suicide on the nightshift years back. Some of the security guards had reported seeing the man and having trouble with alarms as well.

I told my supervisor to take me off warehouse duty. That kind of heart attack wasn't worth the overtime pay.

--T.W.

Nebraska

Deep Breaths

The oddest case I've ever seen in my line of work was this story. A man in his mid-40s arrived at the ER with complaints of shortness of breath, coughing, and chest pressure. Routine scans showed an obstruction in the man's lungs.

This patient did not smoke, nor had he ever. He had a relatively healthy background, exercised daily, and other than his complaints, appeared to be doing well.

At first, we thought we were looking at a tumor, but something about the obstruction seemed off.

Our physician ordered the man to have a biopsy completed.

During the procedure, it was noted the mass could be manipulated with the needle, so the patient was admitted for a thoracotomy.

The procedure produced a wad of matted fur, roughly the size of a golf ball.

When questioned, the patient stated he did have several cats, one a long-haired cat who shed constantly. We theorized the patient had been inhaling his cat's fur, and over time, the fur clumped in his lungs.

We are still not quite sure how this occurred.

--A.W.

Utah

<u>Swimming, Swimming, Swimming</u>

I work at a pediatrician's office. Since the office opened in the mid-1980s, there was a large fish tank along the west wall of the waiting room. My employer is a firm believer in reducing the amount of medications prescribed to children and believes in homeopathic meditation methods, fish-watching being a primary source of stress and pain relief. He's always been incredibly particular about his fish, getting excited to introduce another to the tank. Someone told me he paid $10,000 for one of the fish, and I believe it. My boss once mentioned the aquarium alone cost five grand, and that was when he purchased it in the nineties.

One day, we were having one heck of a time. Not only were we busy with children presenting with a summertime cold that had been sweeping through the town, but our air conditioning was also broken. It was the middle of July and the repairman couldn't make it until the end of the day. We had every window and door in the facility open, along with at least a dozen fans set up to create air circulation.

Patients were just as miserable as we were. Children couldn't sit still. Parents were too hot to chase the kids. Bees and birds kept flying inside.

A woman came inside and sat down in a seat in the center of the room. She carried an oversized wicker tote bag. I did not think too much of it at first. However, after ten or fifteen minutes, I approached the woman and asked if she had a child who needed to be seen. She shook her head and said, "This is where the fish are, right?"

I was confused, but I answered, "Uh, yes, we have a tank for patients. It's a proven relaxation technique." I pointed to the tank that she couldn't have possibly missed. It took up most of the wall.

The woman nodded and said, "That's what I've heard."

I began to inform the woman that if she did not have a child to be seen by our doctor, I would need her to leave the office. I tried to do this politely as possible.

The woman said she would leave, so I returned to the receptionist office.

As soon as I sat down behind my glass window, the woman was right in front of me.

She said, "I just want you to know that fish have emotions, too. They don't want to live in confinement."

I replied, "Uh, okay. They're fish, though."

The woman began shouting madly before she lifted a chair over her head and slammed it against the fish tank glass. Mothers snatched up their children and ran to the other side of the room. A patient's mother tried to stop the crazy woman, but the psycho shoved her to the floor. I called 911. My coworkers locked down the receptionist office as we would in an active shooter situation.

With the second slam of the chair to the tank, the glass shattered, and the contents of the 300-gallon aquarium gushed to the waiting room floor. Water splashed frightened patients and families. The sound of decorative rocks and glass crunching filled the air between the screams.

"Fish have emotions," the woman screeched. "You have no right to cage the fish. They deserve to be free. They deserve to live."

Then, as quickly as she had arrived, the woman left. Nobody in our office dared attempt to restrain the woman or block her from leaving. We were all too afraid of what the nutcase would do next.

My coworkers and I scrambled to scoop fish into Tupperware bowls, paper cups, and any empty containers we could find.

The ironic part about the woman's quest to save the fish is that most of them died.

Officers showed up and took reports from all present witnesses, but the woman was never captured or identified.

My boss was distraught over the incident and took a week off work. He decided against replacing the aquarium, and the decision has disappointed several of our returning patients.

--M.T.

Nevada

Wishy Washy

I responded to a 911 call made from inside a car wash bay. The caller stated he and a friend were trapped inside the bay and needed help getting out.

When I arrived on scene, I pushed the button on the bay exterior, the metal garage door opened, and was met by two men sitting on the hood of a damp car. Both men were drugged out of their minds, that was clear.

"What happened, boys?" I asked.

One man told me the two had been on the way to deliver drugs, when they thought they were being followed by undercover officers. The men entered the car wash bay and washed the vehicle to elude the undercover officers. This is apparently when the doors 'just closed on their own.'

I asked the men if I could take a look inside their vehicle, following the drug admission, and I found about $10,000 worth of meth in the backseat.

Back at the station, with the two dummies in lockup, we reviewed footage obtained from the car wash. The footage showed the men speeding inside and both entrance and exit doors closed, as normal. We watched the men wash their vehicle. Then they tugged at the doors in an attempt to escape. They tugged at the doors for half an hour. When the men accepted they were stuck, we watched them use from their backseat stash and then make the 911 call.

This all could have been solved if the men had pushed the button labeled 'Automatic Door Opener.'

They weren't stuck at all, they were just stupid.

By the way, there were no undercover cops on their tail.

--L.H.

Iowa

The most dedicated woman I've seen in this line of work was the doctor who came in to deliver a baby while she was wearing her wedding dress. She delivered the baby (while layered in multiple blue gowns to protect her dress), congratulated the happy parents, and rushed to the church to continue her delayed wedding ceremony.

--T.S.

Maine

<u>Zombie</u>

In our ER, we usually have two physicians on duty per shift.

One night, we received several MVA victims, following a nasty highway pileup. Unfortunately, Dr. A pronounced an MVA victim as expired. The patient's body was transported to the morgue.

Dr. B went about his business, tending to patients, and reading test results.

About a half hour after the MVA victim was pronounced deceased, another MVA victim from the same crash was walking back from the restroom, which happened to be in the same direction as the morgue.

Dr. B glanced up, stumbled from his chair, and clutched one of the nurse's arms. He was having a heart attack.

When things calmed down, Dr. B confessed that he thought the patient in room four had expired, not the patient in room two. When he saw the patient from room four walking back to our working area, Dr. B panicked.

The story itself is silly, but that night was incredibly hectic for everyone involved. I can't imagine what was running through our doctor's mind when he saw that patient.

--D.L.

Oregon

At an infant's six-week-old wellness check, I (a nurse's assistant) noticed the baby's mother was bottle feeding the newborn chocolate milk.

When I informed the child's mother that it wasn't a good idea to feed her newborn that, mom angrily asked, "Why not? It's milk, isn't it?"

She then told me that she had children ages 2, 3, and 5 at home, so I needed to mind my own business because she 'kept them alive.'

--R.E.

South Carolina

That's Nuts!

On an overnight shift, a patient's wife returned from the snack shop that was across from the cafeteria. She informed me there were squirrels 'running amok' in the cafeteria, and that she had seen them when she peeked in the closed doors. This woman was elderly and we knew that she was not all there, so I dismissed her claims. Who in the world would believe there were squirrels in a hospital cafeteria?

Once the woman's husband was admitted, I finished charting and went to the front to hang out with the registration clerks and our security guards. A call came over the radio, requesting security's immediate response to an 'animal complaint' in the cafeteria.

The elderly woman's complaint was accurate. Squirrels nesting in a vent above the cafeteria had somehow made their way inside the hospital. They ransacked the cafeteria and the kitchen. We all went down to check out the damage once animal control set traps and drove the rest of the animals out of the building.

The squirrels had ripped straws out of the dispensers, emptied the soft drink fountain ice machine, shredded packets of ketchup and tartar sauce, and relieved themselves all over the room. In the kitchen, bags of potatoes and onions were torn open. Half-eaten vegetables were scattered all over the floor. Pots and pans had been knocked from their racks. We're not sure how the animals managed this, but they opened one of the refrigerators and clawed open bags of pre-beaten eggs, spilled pre-cut tomatoes, peppers, and other fruits and vegetables, poked holes in four gallons of milk, and broke the light bulb. There was flour dusting the entire kitchen, with little squirrel tracks throughout the white powder. It was a total disaster.

Obviously, the hospital could not serve meals under those conditions, so the CEO of the hospital ordered that the kitchen and cafeteria remained closed until a professional cleanup crew could enter and disinfect the rooms. Breakfast, lunch, and dinner were catered to the hospital for patients and staff. Families were given vouchers to fast food places and local mom and pop restaurants who were willing to cut a deal with the hospital in exchange for donations or free advertising.

We heard the 'Great Squirrel Fiasco of 2015' cost the hospital more than $15,000 in cleanup, outside sourcing, and the cost of meal vouchers. This cost did not include animal control's fee or the fee to properly remove the nest from the vent system, which also was in need of repair, after maintenance discovered the squirrels created holes in the vents.

--T.U.

Kansas

Police tip #859292507:

If you are on the run, have several warrants for your arrest, and want to antagonize the cops by posting on Facebook 'LOL, I'm never gonna be arrested,' don't tag your current hideout in your post.

That's right. Our perp tagged us and his current location in his status. Facebook even provided a photo of a map for us, with the location marked with a tiny red house icon.

He was arrested 15 minutes after he posted the update.

--Initials and location withheld at request

<u>Surrender</u>

Dispatch notified my partner and me that we needed to respond to a residential burglary. She warned us the burglary was also a medical call, and that EMS could possibly beat us to the residence.

When we arrived on scene, EMS was administering epinephrine to a man with swollen eyes, lips, and a tongue so big you'd think it belonged to a cow.

Medics stated the patient required medical transport, so we tailed them to the emergency room. En route, we contacted dispatch and asked her to explain exactly what the caller had stated on the 911 call.

Our idiot caller broke into a house and was in the process of robbing the homeowners blind, when a bee stung him. The patient/subject then called 911 and confessed to his crimes, only after explaining that he was allergic to bees and had left his epi-pen at home.

We discovered the subject was wanted in connection to other local crimes, including armed robbery.

Following an overnight hospitalization, the criminal was promptly hauled to jail.

--N.S.

Missouri

In a level of stupid that jumped right up to the top of the list of 'Every Stupid Thing I've Seen a Patient Do,' my patient explained that the dates, cities, and states tattooed on his forearms were locations in which he had committed rapes and assaults against women. I slipped out of the room and called the police. My patient was wanted in eight states.

--Initials and location withheld at request

That's Nasty

I work as a registration clerk in emergency services.

One night, a woman and her boyfriend came in. The man complained of full body pain after he 'accidentally' walked off a roof and landed in a shallow kiddie pool. I had seen him before, and I knew he had a history of performing stupid stunts, which he recorded and uploaded to social media.

As I was registering the patient, he picked his nose and ate his boogers. He did not seem embarrassed that he did so whatsoever. I thought his behavior was rather disgusting.

While the patient was in triage, he continuously passed gas, with no apologies to those around him. This, too, I found to be gross.

When I went to his room to verify insurance information, the patient stuck his hand down his pants to adjust his manhood. He then used my pen with the same hand, and he kept trying to touch me when I showed him where to sign on forms. I allowed him to keep the pen, and I used hand sanitizer while I was still in the room, almost as a jab to show him what hygiene looked like.

What really took the cake here was what his girlfriend did. As I was explaining the insurance claim process, the guy's girlfriend, who was lying in bed with him, scraped a scab from the man's face. As if that was not disturbing enough, what she did next caused my stomach to turn.

She ate the scab.

Yes, she *ate* the scab she had just picked off her boyfriend's face. The place where she had plucked it from was bleeding, and the patient just wiped the trickle of blood away with his fingertip. He continued asking me questions as if nothing had happened, even though I kept glancing at his girlfriend and back to him with huge, surprised eyes and an expression of pure horror.

I have never been so repulsed. I couldn't even eat on my lunch break because that scene replayed in my mind repeatedly, and my stomach just couldn't handle digestion at that point.

I mean, can we say, 'Ew?'

--N.K.

Ohio

Caught

Our CEO called mandatory meetings for each shift over the course of a week. All hospital employees were required to attend, so those who were on leave of any kind received notifications requesting they set up individual HR meeting times to discuss key notes of the meetings held in the facility's auditorium.

Everyone knew medications were missing from the pharmacy and ER supply room. Of course, the ones noticed missing first were meds like Dilaudid and Oxy, but after multiple inventories, it was discovered bulk-size bottles of NSAIDs were also missing. This had apparently been going on for months and it was rumored that law enforcement and state officials would soon be visiting the hospital.

Over time, we received emails and fliers that encouraged us to report one another for any sort of suspicious activity. This resulted in many of my coworkers getting in trouble for having affairs or sneaking off to watch porn in the bathroom because others reported these people for 'suspicious disappearances' during work hours.

We were all paranoid. Even people who weren't doing anything wrong were getting reported. I was even reported, but all I was doing was going to my car to eat lunch I had packed in a cooler, because my coworkers kept eating the food I put in the fridge.

The meeting was boring, and after a nightshift, everyone in the audience was tired. We had to watch HR members perform scenarios and then ask us if we should have reported 'Becky' for sneaking a roll of toilet paper home in her purse, like any of us would report a 'Becky' for wanting to wipe her butt. You do what you have to do.

Anyway, about an hour after the meeting started, the CEO was at the podium, reading Power Point slides word for word. His laptop was connected to a projector, and he kept walking in front of the projector screen, but I don't think many people cared, anyway.

Out of the blue, the CEO received an email. Though the notification was a small rectangle in the corner of the screen, the subject read, 'Are we still on for those hydros?' The first line of the email was, 'You still want $400, right?'

Two hundred people in the room, including HR staff, witnessed the email notification. The CEO frantically attempted to click out of the notification and scrambled to explain that the email was 'just a joke.'

He was arrested on felony charges.

--Initials and location withheld at request

A man tried to pay his ED copay with a check. He asked if he could write it over the balance due and receive cash back. We don't usually do this, but since we had just received a device that scanned the check and removed the amount like running a debit card, I did not see that this would matter.

The amount of the man's copay? $50.

The amount he wrote on the check? $242,000.

It was a counterfeit check, too, which landed him in hot water.

Go big or go home, I guess.

--P.S.

Hawaii

<u>Heartbreaking</u>

I am a traveling physician contracted at emergency rooms across the United States. There's not much I haven't witnessed, but one patient's story impacted my life so much that I wanted to share it.

My last patient of the night was a male, 19, who presented with joint pain and muscle aches, sore throat, full body rash, and headaches he rated 10/10 on the pain scale. After reviewing his information, I initially suspected influenza, but that would not explain the full body rash. He was not febrile.

I explained to the patient that we would run tests, including tests to detect STDs.

My patient was admitted to our department for five hours and received fluids while we awaited his lab results.

When I read his results, I struggled with how to deliver the news. After a few minutes of self-deliberation, I entered the room and gently broke the news to the young man that his test results read HIV positive. I explained that I wanted the young man to make a follow up appointment with the hospital lab for another test, and we discussed speaking to his sexual partner(s).

The young man cried and explained he had only one sexual partner, his boyfriend. The two had been dating since the patient was sixteen. He believed his boyfriend had been faithful.

What was disheartening about this, more so, was that the patient stated he and his boyfriend did not use prophylactics. He stated he did not know he needed to use a condom during sex because neither he nor his boyfriend could become pregnant.

In all my years of practicing medicine, I had never heard this from a patient. It hit hard for me, as I am a gay male. I could easily understand how the patient had been miseducated on the necessity of condoms during intercourse because of the reason stated, but it deeply saddened me to think of how others could be facing the same predicament.

Knowing the patient contracted HIV and from a partner he believed to be faithful left me feeling broken inside for months.

--Initials and location withheld at request

Me (Triage) to patient: Are you sexually active?

Patient: Yes.

Patient's husband: *Scoffs* Oh, no you're not. You just lie there like a cold fish and make me do all the work.

--J.D.

Virginia

A Message to Readers

    Hello, everyone! I'm sure you noticed the drastic price change on this title. I wanted to try something new by releasing a 99-cent condensed edition of medical stories. This is not so much a business decision as it is a personal decision. As many of you are aware, I have been working nonstop on a YA novel (young adult) for months. When I'm working, I'm usually neglecting a healthy sleep schedule, and my house becomes a disaster zone. I wanted to satisfy my need to write and your requests for another medical comedy, yet still allow myself time to finish edits on my YA prior to its release, as well as catch up on personal responsibilities. There is a chance I may go against advice and lower the prices on my previous editions of this new series, depending on how this venture turns out.

Choosing submissions for this edition was difficult. Unfortunately, we are bombarded with so many negative news stories these days, and I decided against using several of my submissions because they were too painful for the series. I am extremely grateful to have received submissions from a vast selection of healthcare professionals and first responders.

As usual, I thank you all for your continued support. I've had the joy of interacting with some of you through social media, and I've loved every minute of it. If you have not checked out my social media pages, please know I moderate all pages personally, so if you ever have comments, questions, or concerns, I'll do my best to respond to you.

I hope this edition finds you all well. Thanks for reading, and have a wonderful day!

Check me out on Twitter!

https://twitter.com/AuthorKerryHamm

My website:

http://www.authorkerryhamm.com

I'm also on Facebook. Drop a search for Author Kerry Hamm to find my page!

Manufactured by Amazon.ca
Acheson, AB

13120874R00079